INTERMI͏͏ ͏͏ ͏͏ING

FOR HEALTH, FITNESS AND MACROBIOTICS

Don Matesz, M.A., M.S., L.Ac.

INTERMITTENT FASTING

FOR HEALTH, FITNESS AND MACROBIOTICS

Don Matesz, M.A., M.S., L.Ac.

INTEGRITY PRESS
2016

INTERMITTENT FASTING
FOR HEALTH, FITNESS AND MACROBIOTICS

First Edition

Copyright © 2016 Donald A. Matesz

ISBN-13: 978-1533032218

ISBN-10: 1533032211

Front cover photo © Andrey Kuzmin/Shutterstock License

CONTENTS

NOTE TO THE READER

Diet has a powerful effect on health and fitness. If you are seriously ill or on medications, consult a health care provider knowledgable about nutrition and its health effects and about your medications before you make any changes to your diet or exercise program. You remain always responsible for your choices, actions, and their consequences. This book serves as educational information only and does not substitute for the guidance of a health care professional familiar with your unique situation. Nothing herein is to be construed as a diagnosis or treatment plan for any individual's unique physical condition.

1 WHY FAST?

Everyone goes without eating some part of every day, many wild animals spend days fasting, and we know that people living previous to the modern industrial age fasted for longer periods of time and more often than most people do today. From time immemorial people have used fasting as a means to improve physical health and advance spiritual development.

Due to daily and seasonal fluctuations in wild food supplies, as well as absence of artificial lighting, many mammals, including anthropoid apes and preagricultural humans, eat less often and fast more frequently than modern people and domesticated animals. Mammals including humans have specific metabolic adaptations to regularly going extended periods without food:

> "The ability to function at a high level, both physically and mentally, during extended periods without food may have been of fundamental importance in our evolutionary history. Many adaptations to periodic reductions of food supply are conserved among mammals, including organs for the uptake and storage of rapidly mobilizable glucose (liver glycogen stores) and longer-lasting energy substrates, such as fatty acids in adipose tissue." [1]

Frequent feeding is out out of synch with our biology, contributing to the development of disorders such as obesity,

---

[1] Mattson MP, Allison DB, Fontana L, et al., "Meal frequency and timing in health and disease," *Proceedings of the National Academy of Sciences of the United States of America*. 2014;111(47):16647-16653. <http://www.ncbi.nlm.nih.gov/pmc/articles/PMC4250148/>

metabolic syndrome and non-insulin dependent diabetes mellitus which represent the body's attempt to cope with too frequent and excess food intake.

Because they did not have refrigerators or restaurants, our ancestors could not eat three meals daily. Modern hunter-gatherers generally spent their mornings and early afternoons foraging for foods, then trekked back to home base to prepare the day's one or two main meal(s). This means that they fasted for 16-20 hours daily.

Those human ancestors who had plenty of energy for gathering food during a prolonged daily fast of this sort thrived and left more children than those who couldn't move unless they had food in their stomachs. You are one of the descendants of those people who were well-adapted to being active on an empty stomach.

Among traditional horticulturalists and agriculturalists, adults didn't eat much if anything until after spending the morning and/or early afternoon doing farm or kitchen chores (preparing the first meal from scratch). The English word "dinner" comes from the Old French *disner* which originally meant "breakfast," that is, the meal that comes after the extended daily fast. In French and English "dinner" traditionally referred to the main meal of the day, which in pre-industrial times was taken sometime between late morning and midday. The second, smaller meal was supper, usually taken well before sunset. The word "lunch" originally meant "hunk of bread" and referred to an afternoon snack – not a full meal – had between the first (midday) meal and supper. Only the wealthy, overfed aristocrats ate more than two main meals daily, and they were most prone to obesity, gout, and other diseases.

Ancient people placed great importance on fasting as means of arousing dreams, visions, or ecstasy. In shamanic cultures, shamans and in many cases youths on the verge of adulthood practiced fasting as preparation for their interior journeys to the spirit world to obtain guidance through visions.[2] Most religious traditions – including Islam, Christianity, Judaism, Jainism, Buddhism, Taoism, and Hinduism – suggest some type of fasting as a method of spiritual expression or development.

In ancient Greece, it was believed that eating risked entry of demonic beings that caused disease and shortened life.[3] As in shamanic cultures, among the Greeks fasting was required to prepare for many rituals by which someone sought guidance from spiritual entities. Pythagoras, Abaris, and Epimenides all recommended fasting.

In the Biblical Old Testament, fasting was regarded as a powerful and prayerful preparation for divine revelations. The New Testament depicts the legendary Jesus undertaking a 40 day fast in the desert, during which he has visions, obtains revelations, and develops his spiritual power.

Many members of the modern Seventh-Day Adventist Christian sect follow the advice of the church's founder, Ellen White, to eat only two meals daily – morning and afternoon – and thus have longer daily fasts (16-18 hours). Members of the modern Church of Latter Day Saints (Mormons) are encouraged to do an absolute fast for 24

---

[2] Harner M, *The Way of the Shaman* (HarperOne, 1990).

[3] Kerndt PR, Naughton JL, Driscoll CE, Loxterkamp DA, "Fasting: The History, Pathophysiology and Complications," *Western Journal of Medicine*. 1982;137(5):379-399.
<http://www.ncbi.nlm.nih.gov/pmc/articles/PMC1274154/?page=3>

hours at least once monthly, starting from the age of 8 years old.

According to the Kitagiri Sutta of the Majjhima Nikaya, the legendary Gautama the Buddha recommended that his followers restrict themselves to two meals daily, taken in morning and at mid-day – today called time-restricted feeding – as a method for establishing good health:

> "I, monks, abstain from the night-time meal. As I abstaining from the night-time meal, I sense next-to-no illness, next-to-no affliction, lightness, strength, and a comfortable abiding. Come now. You too abstain from the night-time meal. As you are abstaining from the night-time meal, you, too, will sense next-to-no illness, next-to-no affliction, lightness, strength, and a comfortable abiding." [4]

Since at least 200 B.C., Chinese Taoists have practiced fasting and food restriction as a means of health and spiritual cultivation and to secure immortality.[5] Some ancient Chinese artists practiced fasting to purify their minds and grasp a vision for their artistic expression. According to some legends, Bodhidharma, a patriarch of Chinese chán (zen) Buddhism, practiced limited fasting during his quest for spiritual awakening.[6]

---

[4] Kitagiri Sutta: At Kitagiri. Trans. by Thanissaro Bhikkhu, 2005. <http://www.accesstoinsight.org/tipitaka/mn/mn.070.than.html>

[5] Eisen M, "Chinese Bigu for Yang Sheng," *Yang Sheng* 2011 October 15. <http://yang-sheng.com/?p=3874>

[6] Ibid.

Today we know that periods of complete fasting (no food at all) of sufficient duration elicit beneficial metabolic states in the brain and heart. It is possible that these metabolic states may help an individual to elicit states of consciousness that contribute to insight and spiritual development.

In summary, it seems that in traditional cultures most people spent 16 to 20 hours daily in the fasted (yang) state and only 4 to 8 hours in the fed (yin) state whereas modern people spend more like 12 to 16 hours in the fed (yin) state, and only 8 to 12 hours in the fasted (yang) state. In addition, fasting was considered a reliable method for increasing one's lifespan and access to spiritual insight.

Modern people feed too often, and fast too little. This means they are full more often than they are empty. This can happen even among people who eat a proper, plant-based diet. Eating too often and fasting too little inevitably results in accumulations of excess nutriment and waste in the body, which promotes disease. It may also make our minds dull, insensitive, and less capable of experiencing the full range of higher, insightful states of consciousness described by shamans and seekers throughout time.

2 DEGREES OF FASTING

Historically the word "fasting" has referred to any voluntary reduction of or abstinence from some or all food or nutritive beverages or both for a period of time. An absolute fast consists of abstaining from all nutritive food and beverages other than water for a specific period of time.

Chronic calorie restriction (CR) is an example of limited fasting, in which one or more types of food are restricted on a continuous daily basis, resulting in a substantial (20-40%) reduction of energy (calorie) intake, but without a change in meal frequency (number and timing of daily meals). Popular examples include conventional dieting, and some types of religious fasting that restrict specific foods but not others, including the Biblical Daniel Fast and the Greek Orthodox fasting rituals (discussed below in Mediterranean Fasting). The CR Society International promotes chronic calorie restriction with optimal nutrition (CRON) as a path to longevity.

Periodic or intermittent absolute fasting – also known as water fasting – involves incorporating into one's diet regular periods of 16-36 hours wherein one does not consume any food or nutritive beverages. There exist two common strategies for intermittent fasting for health benefits. One involves fasting for about 24 hours once or twice weekly, perhaps occasionally for longer periods of time.

Another approach involves limiting daily intake of food and nutritive beverages to a specific time window – e.g. 1-8 hours - hence producing periods of absolute fasting for 16-23 hours daily. This is sometimes called time-restricted feeding (TRF). As already noted, this was the normal way of eating for non-agricultural people, likely normal for most of humanity prior to the industrial age, and advocated by the legendary Gautama the Buddha. It is also a common practice of present-day Seventh Day Adventists (discussed below).

Some people have used the term "intermittent fasting" to refer to both periodic absolute fasting and time-restricted feeding. However, the word "intermittent" means "occurring at irregular intervals." Since people use absolute fasting and time-restricted feeding at more or less regular intervals such as once or twice weekly for absolute fasting and daily for time-restricted feeding , and "periodic" means "recurring at intervals of time," I think it is more appropriate to describe them as periodic fasting methods.

As noted, the CR Society International promotes chronic calorie-restriction with optimal nutrition (CRON) as a path to longevity. There exists considerable evidence that chronic caloric restriction delays aging and prolongs lifespan in non-primate animals. A 23-year study found that caloric restriction alone did reduce disease risks and reduce the rate of aging, but did not extend the lives of rhesus monkeys.[7] However, chronic caloric restriction may mean chronic hunger, preoccupation with food, physical wasting, and loss of libido.

---

[7] NIH. "Calorie Restriction May Not Extend Life," *NIH Research Matters* 2012 September 17. . <https://www.nih.gov/news-events/nih-research-matters/calorie-restriction-may-not-extend-life>

Some evidence suggests that the benefits of caloric restriction are due primarily to restriction of intake of protein,[8, 9, 10] or, more specifically, the amino acids leucine and methionine. It appears that the benefit of protein restriction comes about largely through a reduction of excessive IGF-1 levels. One can easily achieve protein, leucine and methionine restriction and reduced IGF-1 levels without enduring chronic hunger or protein deficiency by consuming a whole foods plant-based diet, because animal foods are the principal sources of excess calories, protein, leucine, and methionine. Studies in humans indicate that strictly plant-based diets with low but sufficient protein contents and adequate calories reduce IGF-1 levels more than calorically restricted diets that contain animal

---

[8] Nakagawa S, Lagisz M, Hector KL, Spencer HG, "Comparative and meta-analytic insights into life extension via dietary restriction," *Aging Cell*. 2012 Jun;11(3):401-9.
<http://onlinelibrary.wiley.com/doi/10.1111/j.1474-9726.2012.00798.x/epdf>

[9] Gallinetti J, Harputlugil E, Mitchell JR, "Amino acid sensing in dietary-restriction-mediated longevity: roles of signal-transducing kinases GCN2 and TOR," *The Biochemical journal* 2013;449(1):1-10. doi:10.1042/BJ20121098.
<http://www.ncbi.nlm.nih.gov/pmc/articles/PMC3695616/>

[10] Levine ME, Suarez JA, Brandhorst S, et al., "Low Protein Intake is Associated with a Major Reduction in IGF-1, Cancer, and Overall Mortality in the 65 and Younger but Not Older Population," *Cell metabolism* 2014;19(3):407-417. doi:10.1016/j.cmet.2014.02.006.
<https://www.ncbi.nlm.nih.gov/pmc/articles/PMC3988204/>

protein.[11, 12] Moreover, it has been found that people aged 50-65 who consume a high animal protein intake (20% of energy or more) had a 75% increase in total mortality, a 4-fold increase in cancer and a 73-fold increase in diabetes mortality during an 18 year observation period.[13] In that same study, a "moderate" protein intake (10-19% of energy) was associated with a 23-fold increased risk in death from diabetes and a 3-fold increased risk of death from cancer. Protein from plants was not associated with increased mortality. Restriction of intake of the branch-chained amino acids –leucine, isoleucine, and valine – improves metabolic health in humans.[14] Animal proteins provide much higher levels of these amino acids than plant proteins.

[11] Fontana L, Partridge L, Longo VD, "Dietary Restriction, Growth Factors and Aging: from yeast to humans," *Science (New York, NY)*. 2010;328(5976):321-326. doi:10.1126/science.1172539. <http://www.ncbi.nlm.nih.gov/pmc/articles/PMC3607354/>

[12] Fontana L, Weiss EP, Villareal DT, Klein S, Holloszy JO, "Long-term effects of calorie or protein restriction on serum IGF-1 and IGFBP-3 concentration in humans," *Aging Cell*. 2008;7(5):681-687. doi:10.1111/j.1474-9726.2008.00417.x. <http://www.ncbi.nlm.nih.gov/pmc/articles/PMC2673798/>

[13] Levine ME, et al., op. cit.

[14] Fontana L, Cummings NE, Arriola Apelo SI, et al., "Decreased consumption of branched chain amino acids improves metabolic health," *Cell reports*. 2016;16(2):520-530. doi:10.1016/j.celrep.2016.05.092. <https://www.ncbi.nlm.nih.gov/pmc/articles/PMC4947548/>

Some may consider a whole foods plant-based macrobiotic diet a type of food restriction fasting because it restricts or removes all animal products and refined plant foods (sugar, processed starches, processed proteins, oils). ESSENTIAL MACROBIOTICS and THE MACROBIOTIC ACTION PLAN cover the principles and practical implementation of a healthy whole foods plant-based macrobiotic diet.

In this booklet, you will learn the benefits of implementing periodic 16-24 hour absolute fasts and time-restricted feeding to enhance the benefits of a whole foods plant-based macrobiotic diet, which may or may not be restricted in energy (caloric) content, depending on your goals (weight loss, weight maintenance, weight gain).

If you have a goal of weight loss, periodic fasting can help you more easily achieve fat loss without loss of lean tissue. If you have a goal of weight maintenance, periodic fasting can help you maintain a lean condition without being obsessive about control of energy, fat, or carbohydrate intake when you eat meals.

If you have a goal to gain some lean muscle tissue, periodic fasting can help you prevent gaining fat as your weight increases.

Meanwhile, a whole foods strictly plant-based diet that includes regular periodic fasting may have the same or superior overall health and longevity benefits as chronic caloric restriction without the undesirable side effects of chronic energy deprivation. Thus, periodic fasting can help you create a great life (*macro-bios*).

3 MEDITERRANEAN LIMITED FASTING

By now, many people have heard that the Mediterranean diet confers health benefits. This idea came from studies of the people of Crete, done in the mid-20th century, which found that at that time, people living the traditional lifestyle of Crete had low rates of cardiovascular disease and cancer and greater longevity than any other nation known at the time.

Scientists and science writers in the media have attributed the excellent health of the Cretan people to various foods found in their diet, such as olive oil, grapes and grape products (such as wine), whole grains, seafoods, walnuts, purslane, and others. These all may play some role in the "Mediterranean effect," and people may find it easy to add these foods to their diets, but the benefits of the Cretan diet may lie largely in the combination of food restriction fasting – consisting of quite limited intake of animal foods along with restrictions on olive oil intake – that results in significant caloric reductions in the context of a whole foods plant-based diet.

The traditional Cretan diet was composed primarily of bread, potatoes, legumes, vegetables and fruits, and meat, poultry, fish, eggs and dairy products provided only about 7 percent of total kcalorie intake.[15]

If you didn't know that fasting and food restrictions played an important role in the traditional, health-giving "Mediterranean" diet, I don't feel surprised. I have not seen

---

[15] Renaud S, de Lorgeril M, Delaye J, et al., "Cretan Mediterranean diet for prevention of coronary heart disease," *Am J Clin Nutr*. 1995 Jun;61(6 Suppl):1360S-1367S. PubMed PMID: 7754988.

a single popular report on the Mediterranean effect or diet that made any reference to fasting or caloric restriction.

But limited "fasting" resulting in significant caloric restriction played a very significant role in the traditional diet of Crete's people in times up to the mid-20th century when they were noted for their health and longevity.[16] A majority of people on Crete belonged to the Greek Orthodox Christian Church (GOC). This Church prescribes a total of 180–200 days of "fasting"—here meaning abstention from certain foods--per year. Faithful church members avoid olive oil, meat, fish, milk and dairy products every Wednesday and Friday throughout the year. In addition, the Church specifies three principal fasting periods per year:

i) A total of 40 days preceding Christmas during which the Church advises abstention from meat, dairy products and eggs, while it allows fish and olive oil except on Wednesdays and Fridays.

ii) A period of 48 days preceding Easter (Lent), during which fasters eat fish on only two days and olive oil only on weekends, and avoid meat, dairy products and eggs on all days.

iii) A total of 15 days in August (the Assumption) having the same dietary rules apply as for Lent with the exception that this period allows fish consumption only on August 6th.

---

[16] Sarri KO, Linardakis MK, Bervanaki FN, et al., "Greek Orthodox fasting rituals: a hidden characteristic of the Mediterranean diet of Crete," *Br J Nutr*. 2004 Aug;92(2):277-84. PubMed PMID: 15333159.

Orthodox fasting rituals allow seafood such as shrimps, squid, cuttlefish, octopus, lobsters, crabs as well as snails on all fasting days throughout the year.[17]

One interesting note here, on the many of the "fast" days the faithful abstained from olive oil, the food that nevertheless has for some become synonymous with Mediterranean diet. Many people think they will get the good health of the people of Crete by eating more olive oil, but looking at the people on Crete, it is more likely their good health comes from the caloric restriction that results from avoiding olive oil on a great many days of the year.

Greek Orthodox fasting rituals produce caloric restriction on half of the days of the year. One study showed that people on Crete who followed the fasting rules of the GOC had, at the end of the food restriction periods, average caloric intakes of only about 1600 kcalories, almost 22% lower than Cretans who did not follow the "fasting" rules. These Mediterranean "fasters" have an average caloric intake at least 30% lower than typical Americans eating 2400 or more calories daily.

Although Greek Orthodox "fasting" does not necessarily involve prolonged periods without any food intake at all, it does result in significant caloric restriction, which allows the body to clear itself of accumulations of potentially hazardous excess nutrients (e.g. stored fat) and metabolic waste products. As discussed below, it appears that reduction of feeding frequency can reduce caloric intake, and has benefits similar to caloric restriction even if total energy intake does not decline.

---

[17] Sarri KO, Tzanakis NE, Linardakis MK, et al., "Effects of Greek orthodox christian church fasting on serum lipids and obesity," *BMC Public Health* 2003;3:16.
<http://www.ncbi.nlm.nih.gov/pmc/articles/PMC156653/>

4 SEVENTH DAY ADVENTIST FASTING

Seventh Day Adventists (SDAs) living in California have an average life expectancy about 9-10 years longer than non-SDA Californians.[18] Since vegan and vegetarian SDAs live longer than non-vegetarian SDAs, many researchers have tended to exclusively credit abstention from animal foods for this greater lifespan.

While a large body of evidence from the Adventist Health Study indicates that limitation of animal foods does play a large role in Adventist health and longevity, there is another factor in play. The dietary guidelines of the SDA church include the suggestion to eat only two meals daily, which results in longer daily fasting periods than typical among non-SDA people.[19]

The founder of the SDA church, Ellen G. White, wrote:

> "The stomach must have careful attention. It must not be kept in continual operation. Give this misused and much-abused organ some peace and quiet and rest. After the stomach has done its work for one meal, do not crowd more work upon it before it has had a chance to rest and before a sufficient supply of gastric juice is provided by nature to care for more food. Five hours at least should

[18] Fraser GE, Shavlik DJ, "Ten Years of Life: Is It a Matter of Choice?," *Arch Intern Med*. 2001;161(13):1645-1652. doi:10.1001/archinte.161.13.1645. <http://archinte.jamanetwork.com/article.aspx?articleid=648593>

[19] Kelly CJ, "A controlled trial of reduced meal frequency without caloric restriction in healthy, normal-weight, middle-aged adults," *Am J Clin Nutr* 2007 Oct; 86(4): 1254-1255. <http://ajcn.nutrition.org/content/86/4/1254.2.long>

elapse between each meal, and always bear in mind that if you would give it a trial, you would find that two meals are better than three." [20]

White also recommended avoiding eating before sleeping and making breakfast – the first meal of the day, whenever it is taken – the most substantial meal.

"Another pernicious habit is that of eating just before bed-time. The regular meals may have been taken; but because there is a sense of faintness, more food is eaten. By indulgence, this wrong practice becomes a habit, and often so firmly fixed that it is thought impossible to sleep without food. As a result of eating late suppers, the digestive process is continued through the sleeping hours. But though the stomach works constantly, its work is not properly accomplished. The sleep is often disturbed with unpleasant dreams, and in the morning the person awakes unrefreshed, and with little relish for breakfast. When we lie down to rest, the stomach should have its work all done, that it, as well as the other organs of the body, may enjoy rest. For persons of sedentary habits, late suppers are particularly harmful. With them the disturbance created is often the beginning of disease that ends in death." [21]

"It is the custom and order of society to take a slight breakfast. But this is not the best way to treat the

---

[20] White EG. *Ellen G. White Writings*, Letter 73a, 1896. <https://text.egwwritings.org/publication.php?pubtype=Book&bookCode=CD&pagenumber=173>

[21] White EG. *Ellen G. White Writings*, The Ministry of Healing, 303-304. <https://text.egwwritings.org/publication.php?pubtype=Book&bookCode=TSDF&pagenumber=38>

stomach. At breakfast time the stomach is in a better condition to take care of more food than at the second or third meal of the day. The habit of eating a sparing breakfast and a large dinner is wrong. Make your breakfast correspond more nearly to the heartiest meal of the day." [22]

White's advice has been supported by scientific research. People assigned to consume most of their calories early in the day (700 kcal breakfast, 500 kcal lunch, 200 kcal supper) showed less hunger, greater satiety, and greater reductions of body weight, waist circumference, serum triglycerides, fasting glucose, fasting insulin, and insulin resistance than those assigned to eat most of their food late in the day (200 kcal breakfast, 500 kcal lunch, 700 kcal dinner) for 12 weeks.[23] Some research indicates that animals and people who consume most of their food late in their normal waking period have greater body fat and more metabolic disorders than those who consume most of their food early in the

---

[22] White EG. *Ellen G. White Writings* Letter 3, 1884.
<https://text.egwwritings.org/publication.php?pubtype=Book&bookCode=CD&pagenumber=173>

[23] Jakubowicz D, Barnea M, et al., "High Caloric intake at breakfast vs. dinner differentially influences weight loss of overweight and obese women," *Obesity* 2013 Dec;21(12);2504-2512.
<http://onlinelibrary.wiley.com/doi/10.1002/oby.20460/full>

normal waking period (i.e. early in daylight hours for humans).[24, 25] I discuss this further in chapter 9.

Typically, SDAs who implement the two-meal plan eat breakfast and lunch. This pattern is also recommended by Chinese medicine, which acknowledges greater digestive efficiency in the morning and noon hours, but greater storage efficiency in the evening hours.

Assuming these two meals occur within about 4 to 8 hours of each other, this would result in daily fasting periods of 16 to 20 hours. This time-restricted feeding (TRF) regimen very likely contributes to the exceptional health and longevity of Adventists.

---

[24] Ibid.

[25] Fuse Y, Hirao A, Kuroda H, et al., "Differential roles of breakfast only (one meal per day) and a bigger breakfast with a small dinner (two meals per day) in mice fed a high-fat diet with regard to induced obesity and lipid metabolism," *Journal of Circadian Rhythms*, 10, p.Art. 4. DOI: http://doi.org/10.1186/1740-3391-10-4 <http://www.jcircadianrhythms.com/articles/10.1186/1740-3391-10-4/>

5 FEEDING & FASTING: YIN & YANG

In the universal scientific theory of Taoism, the terms yin and yang[26] simply represent two types of phenomena presented in our experience. Applied as a medical theory, every physiological disorder results from an imbalance between yin and yang influences.

Simply put, phenomena which we experience as relatively cool, quiet, slow, dark, and moist belong to the yin category, and those which we experience as relatively warm, loud, fast, bright, and dry belong to the yang category. The classic yin-yang symbol graphically depicts the two poles of phenomena. In this symbol, yang is represented by the white domains, and yin by the black domains.

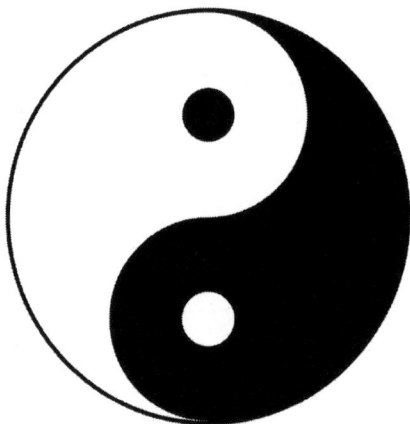

When the body has too much exposure to yin influences and not enough to yang influences, it becomes too yin itself; and

---

[26] Properly pronounced "yeen" and "yahng."

vice versa, when it has too much exposure to yang influences and not enough to yin, it becomes too yang. Food is moist and material, so feeding produces a more yin condition, whereas fasting and exercise burn up food and discharge fluids (through sweating) so they produce a more yang condition.

This is confirmed by Western physiology, which reports that in the fed state the body shifts into a rest-and-digest mode of accumulating matter and energy that is ruled by the parasympathetic nervous system. Feeding stimulates the pancreas to release the hormone insulin, which drives sugar, amino acids, and fatty acids out of the blood into cells, and stimulates the build-up (expansion) of glycogen, protein, and fat stores. After meals the body tends to feel heavy and lethargic, the mind is more dull, and there is a natural tendency to sleepiness.

In the normal fasted state the sympathetic nervous system becomes dominant and the body converts stored matter to energy. During a fast the pancreas releases the hormone glucagon, which has opposite effects of insulin, stimulating the breakdown of fats and glycogen. Consequently, the body feels lighter and energetic, the mind is more alert, and there is a natural tendency to physical and mental activity. In the fasted state, matter is converted into energy and dispersed outward, which depletes body water and hardens up tissues as glycogen and fat stores contract, so is a net yang process from the standpoint of effect on the material body.

6 PHYSIOLOGY OF FASTING

After a meal, your body shifts into a period of digestion and absorption that lasts for about 3 hours; in this fed state, the body uses the carbohydrates, fat, and proteins from the food to replenish energy stores depleted during fasting or exercise. If glycogen stores have been depleted (by fasting or exercise), carbohydrates will first get stored as glycogen, both in the liver and in the muscles, but if glycogen stores are full, the extra carbohydrate (starch or sugar) will get converted to fat.

From roughly 3 to about 12-18 hours after a meal, your body operates in the "postabsorptive" or "early fasting" state. In the early part of this stage, the body cells derive much of their energy needs from breakdown of stored carbohydrate (glycogen – the bulk of the which was supplied by the last meal) and body fat.

Depending on the size of your last meal, sometime in the period between 12 and 18 hours after that meal you transition to "fasting" metabolism, which continues up to about 48 hours. During this stage, between about 15 and 48 hours past the last meal, your body shifts to getting an increasing proportion of its energy from fat—one of the main goals of the anyone seeking fat loss.

Other major health benefits of fasting also occur in this stage. During this phase you get these benefits (discussed in the next chapter), without incurring major losses of lean healthy tissue (such as muscle), or metabolic power, so long as you get food by the end of 48 hours.

If you go without eating for more than about 72 hours, your metabolism shifts to the "long-term fasting" or "starvation" stage. At this stage, you may start to see losses in lean tissue. I recommend that you generally avoid fasting more than 36 hours, so you get all the benefits of fasting, but never incur the losses involved in starving.

7 BENEFICIAL METABOLIC EFFECTS OF FASTING

Regular moderate-length periods of fasting (15-24 hours) can help you achieve the lean and healthy body you desire, because it has numerous beneficial metabolic effects.

1. Glycogen depletion

When you consume more carbohydrate than immediately needed, the liver and muscles convert the excess into a type of starch called glycogen. The liver can store about 100 g of glycogen, and the muscles 300 to 400 g.

When you fast, the liver store of glycogen gets used up in 8 to 10 hours, and muscle glycogen reduces by about 50 percent in 24 hours. These reductions in glycogen stores cause the body to make metabolic changes that increase the burning of fat.

In fact, since full glycogen stores reduce the body's use of fat as fuel, you must deplete them to activate maximum fat burning. If you exercise intensely during a fast your ratio of energy output to energy intake is maximized at the same time that glycogen is maximally depleted.

Since 16 hours of fasting significantly depletes liver glycogen stores, implementing daily fasts of 14-16 hours will improve your ability to utilize body fat as fuel, and can help you reduce your daily total food energy intake to reduce body fat stores. Alternatively, you can implement a couple of 24 hour fasts each week to achieve the same goals, or combine the two approaches to fit your lifestyle.

2. Increased insulin sensitivity

Research has demonstrated that a 16 hour fast improves insulin sensitivity of muscle cells, which means that when you do eat carbohydrates, they will get channeled more effectively to your muscle cells for use as fuel or to be stored as glycogen, rather than getting channeled to fat cells to get converted to fat.[27] Improving insulin sensitivity is a key goal in preventing and treating type 2 diabetes (NIDDM).

By the end of a 24 hour fast, blood insulin levels drop by about 35%, and over 72 hours, they drop by more than 50%.[28] You want this to happen because insulin stimulates fat storage and blocks fat burning, so reduced insulin levels translates to reduced fat storage and increased fat burning.

Regular fasting also improves insulin sensitivity. After a 15 day period during which subjects fasted 20 hours every alternate day, but ate abundantly on other days and did not lose body fat, insulin sensitivity improved markedly.[29] Insulin insensitivity plays a role in diabetes type 2, so intermittent fasting can help prevent or reverse this disease. Increased insulin sensitivity results in lower insulin production, hence better fat metabolism.

3. Increases in fat-metabolizing enzymes
As you enter a fasted, glycogen-depleted state, your body

---

[27] Heijboer AC, Donga E, Voshol PJ, et al., "Sixteen hours of fasting differentially affects hepatic and muscle insulin sensitivity in mice," *J Lipid Res* 2005;46:582-588.

[28] Klein S, et al., "Progressive Alterations in lipid and glucose metabolism during short-term fasting in young adult men," *Am J Physiology* 1993; 265 (Endocrinology and metabolism 28):E801-E806 <http://ajpendo.physiology.org/content/ajpendo/265/5/E801.full.pdf>

[29] Halberg N, Henriksen M, So¨derhamn N, et al., "Effect of intermittent fasting and refeeding on insulin action in healthy men," *J Appl Physiol* 99:2128-2136, 2005. <http://jap.physiology.org/content/99/6/2128.long>

cells rapidly increase their production of enzymes involved in burning fat. The body fat cells release fat into the blood stream, and the muscle cells—the primary fat burners in the body—start sucking the fat out of the blood stream to burn for fuel.

The muscle cells use an enzyme called uncoupling protein-3 (UCP3) when burning fat. Fifteen hours of fasting raises the level of UCP3 five-fold, and by 40 hours the level has increased by more than 10-fold![30]

At the end of 24 hours of fasting, release of fat from fat cells and use of fat by muscle cells increases by 50%, and most of this increase occurs between 18 and 24 hours. When you fast regularly (once or twice weekly) the body adapts by keeping levels of fat burning enzymes elevated at all times. Periodic fasting literally turns your body into a fat-burning machine.

4. Lipolysis
About 12 to 18 hours into a period of fasting, lipolysis, the breakdown of fat, becomes the major energy pathway. As blood sugar reaches normal fasting levels, the body responds by releasing glucagon and epinephrine (adrenaline), and these hormones act to stimulate the breakdown of fat and increase the cells' use of fat as fuel. The increased levels of epinephrine also give you a sense of mental clarity and energy not available in the fed state without taking drugs like caffeine.

As the cells metabolize fats in the absence of carbohydrate, they convert the fats to ketones, a process called ketosis. Whereas glucose (from starch, sugar, or glycogen) has only 4

---

[30] Tunstall RJ, et al., "Fasting activates the gene expression of UCP3 independent of genes necessary for lipid transport and oxidation in skeletal muscle," *Biochem Biophys Res Comm* 2002; 294:301-308

calories per gram, ketones supply 4.6 calories per gram. In an individual not adapted to fasting, all tissues of the body except for red blood cells and the central nervous tissue can use ketones for fuel. (The brain can adapt to using ketones after prolonged fasting.[31]) During the period between 16 and 36 hours of a fast the body reserves any available glucose for the red blood cells and central nervous system, and adapts to burning ketones in other tissues, so you won't lack energy during brief absolute fasts.

One of the most important ketones has the name ß-hydroxybutyrate (BHB). As noted, as a ketone, BHB releases more energy per gram than glucose. In addition, BHB counteracts neurotoxins capable of causing Parkinson's and Alzheimer's diseases and counters free radical damage.[32, 33]

If you exercise during a fast, your muscle cells will burn fat for fuel at a higher rate than if you exercise in a fed state.

Since fat burning increases dramatically during a fast, even

[31] Owen OE, "Ketone bodies as a fuel for the brain during starvation," *Biochem Mol Biol Educ* 2005 Jul;33(4):246-51. <http://onlinelibrary.wiley.com/doi/10.1002/bmb.2005.49403304246/full>

[32] Tieu K, Perier C, Caspersen C, et al., "D-ß-Hydroxybutyrate rescues mitochondrial respiration and mitigates features of Parkinson disease," *J Clin Invest* 2003;112(6):892-901. doi:10.1172/JCI200318797. <http://www.ncbi.nlm.nih.gov/pmc/articles/PMC193668/>

[33] Kashiwaya Y, Takeshima T, Mori N, et al., "d-ß-Hydroxybutyrate protects neurons in models of Alzheimer's and Parkinson's disease," *Proceedings of the National Academy of Sciences of the United States of America* 2000;97(10):5440-5444. <http://www.ncbi.nlm.nih.gov/pmc/articles/PMC25847/>

without changing the types of foods you eat on non-fasting days, fasting facilitates rapid fat loss. The average largely sedentary person expends 1500 to 2500 calories daily in life maintenance and activities, and one pound of stored fat contains 3500 calories. If the average largely sedentary individual abstains from food for a whole day each week, and eats normally on non-fasting days, he or she can lose one-half to two-thirds of a pound of fat each week; and if this individual fasted two days of each week, he or she could lose at least one pound of fat in the week.

Remember, you can achieve those results just by fasting. If you eat a low fat plant-based diet, you may lose fat even more rapidly.

5. Increased human growth hormone (hGH) release

One of the most remarkable effects of fasting consists of dramatic increases in release of human growth hormone.[34, 35] People presently spend thousands of dollars monthly for injections of growth hormone to reverse the effects of aging, but they could get increased exposure to growth hormone without monetary expense by simply fasting once or twice weekly, or 16-23 hours daily.

The pituitary gland releases GH in pulses throughout the day.

---

[34] Ho KY, Veldhuis JD, Johnson ML, et al., "Fasting enhances growth hormone secretion and amplifies the complex rhythms of growth hormone secretion in man," *Journal of Clinical Investigation* 1988;81(4):968-975.
<http://www.ncbi.nlm.nih.gov/pmc/articles/PMC329619/>

[35] Kerndt PR, Naughton JL, Driscoll CE, Loxterkamp DA, "Fasting: The History, Pathophysiology and Complications." *Western Journal of Medicine* 1982;137(5):379-399.
<http://www.ncbi.nlm.nih.gov/pmc/articles/PMC1274154/>

Fasting for just 24 hours has a dramatic effect on GH output; it increases the frequency of GH pulses by 25%, it doubles the peak amplitude of GH pulses, and it quadruples the interpeak serum GH levels.[36]

Growth hormone stimulates breakdown of fat, growth of muscle, and repair of tissues and DNA. For this reason, regular fasting may make you look and feel younger, lose fat, and build muscle.

An 8 week long study compared the effects on people of eating all caloric requirements in just one as opposed to the conventional three meals per day.[37] This study found that the people assigned to fasting 20 hours daily, then eating all of their caloric requirements in only 1 evening meal each day lost an average of 1.4 kg (3 lb.) body mass and 2.1 kg (4.6 lb.) fat mass over the eight weeks, which means that they gained an average of 1.6 lb. lean mass over the study period, with no change in exercise habits. If not experimental error, this increase in lean mass may have resulted from increased GH output during the long fasting periods daily. The results of this study were supported in a study which found that mice subjected to energy and macronutrient restriction had higher bone density and no age-related loss of muscle mass

---

[36] Ho KY, et al.. Op. cit..

[37] Stote KS, Baer DJ, Spears K, et al., "A controlled trial of reduced meal frequency without caloric restriction in healthy, normal-weight, middle-aged adults," *The Am J Clin Nutr* 2007;85(4):981-988. <http://www.ncbi.nlm.nih.gov/pmc/articles/PMC2645638/>

compared to mice fed ad libitum.[38]

6. Elimination of excess water and sodium

Elevated insulin levels cause your body to retain sodium and water. Fasting lowers your insulin level, and this causes natriuresis, the elimination of sodium, and water, through urination. This relieves edema and eliminates that puffy, doughy appearance you don't like.

7. Healing of gut inflammation and leakage

Diets rich in animal flesh, eggs, or milk, or fats or oils, increase the risk of inflammation of the gut, whereas diets rich in plant food reduce gut inflammation.[39] As this progresses, the gut becomes leaky, allowing incompletely digested nutrients to enter the blood stream. Once these incompletely digested nutrients, particularly animal-source proteins, enter the blood, the white blood cells mount an attack on them, causing inflammation and making you feel sick. Some of the cells make antibodies to the foreign proteins, and if these proteins had any similarity to proteins in your own tissues, the antibodies will proceed to attack your own tissues, causing autoimmune diseases.

Fasting may decrease intestinal permeability (leakage) and thus be beneficial for disorders involving leaky gut such as

---

[38] Van Norren K, Rusli F, van Dijk M, et al., "Behavioural changes are a major contributing factor in the reduction of sarcopenia in caloric-restricted ageing mice," *Journal of Cachexia, Sarcopenia and Muscle* 2015;6(3):253-268. doi:10.1002/jcsm.12024.

[39] Lee D, Albenberg L, Compher C, et al., "Diet in the Pathogenesis and Treatment of Inflammatory Bowel Diseases," *Gastroenterology* 2015;148:1087-1106.

autoimmune diseases.[40]

8. Reduction of oxidative stress and inflammation

Overweight asthma patients who adhered to 8 weeks of alternate day 80% caloric restriction experienced significant sustained decreases in serum levels of several markers of oxidative stress and inflammation,[41] including C-reactive protein (C-RP), interleukin-6 (IL-6), tumor necrosis factor-alpha, ceramides, leptin, and serum brain-derived neurotrophic factor (BDNF). Serum levels of TNF alpha declined by about 60%, BDNF by about 70%.

In this same study, markers of oxidative stress also declined dramatically. Levels of protein carbonyls and 8-isoprostane fell 80%, nitrotyrosine fell more than 90%, and 4-hydroxynonenal adducts fell about 50%.

In addition, studies show that global cell proliferation declines on 24/24 fast/feast programs. This means fasting 24 hours stops the growth of "rogue" cells that could become tumors, cysts, or cancers, and reduces cell proliferation characteristic of atherosclerosis and some other diseases like psoriasis.

---

[40] Sunqvist T, Lindstrom F, Magnusson KE, et al., "Influence of fasting on intestinal permeability and disease activity in patients with rheumatoid arthritis," *Scand J Rheumatol* 1082;11(1):33-8. Abstract.

[41] Johnson J et al, "Alternate day calorie restriction improves clinical findings and reduces markers of oxidative stress and inflammation in overweight adults with moderate asthma," *Free Radic Biol Med* 2007 Mar 1;42(5):665-74. Epub 2006 Dec 14.
<http://www.ncbi.nlm.nih.gov/pmc/articles/PMC1859864/>

9. Central nervous system (CNS) improvements

Fasting improves a number of aspects of brain health and function.[42, 43] It protects brain neurons from stressors, including chemical toxins. While fasting decreases the amount of brain-derived neurotrophic factor in the blood– a good sign–it increases the amount of brain-derived neurotrophic factor where it belongs, in the brain itself, which promotes healthy growth of brain neurons and has an antidepressant effect. Fasting after a brain injury improves recovery. There exists evidence that dietary restriction reduces the negative effects of vitamin or mineral deficiency on the nervous system.[44] Numerous animal studies show that fasting improves learning and delays brain aging. Thus, it is likely that regular periodic fasting will help protect you for neurodegenerative diseases like Alzheimer's dementia and Parkinson's disease.

10. Sensory enhancement

Fasting causes a rapid change in the sensitivity of sensory organs. Frequent feeding dulls the sense organs, especially if one's habitual food has high fat or sugar contents or intense flavoring with salt or spices. After a fast, your sense of taste and appreciation of subtle flavors dramatically improves.

---

[42] Longo VD, Mattson MP, "Fasting: Molecular Mechanisms and Clinical Applications," *Cell metabolism* 2014;19(2):181-192. doi:10.1016/j.cmet.2013.12.008.
<http://www.ncbi.nlm.nih.gov/pmc/articles/PMC3946160/>

[43] Mattson MP, Duan W, Guo Z, "Meal size and frequency affect neuronal plasticity and vulnerability to disease: cellular and molecular mechanisms, *J Neurochem* 2003;84:417-31.
<http://onlinelibrary.wiley.com/doi/10.1046/j.1471-4159.2003.01586.x/epdf>

[44] Ibid.

This helps you to break the addiction to high fat, high sugar, highly seasoned processed foods.

11. Cellular Cleansing

The normal process of metabolism of nutrients produces free radicals, which damage proteins and organelles in our cells, resulting in the effects we associate with aging. This damage particularly affects the mitochondria, the energy-generating organelles in every cell. If the cells don't remove damaged, malfunctioning mitochondria, the latter begin to spew out suicidal proteins prompting the entire cell to die. The aging process consists of this death of cells.

When fasted for 16 or more hours, your cells switch to a self-cleansing mode called *autophagy* where they release enzymes that digest the metabolic waste accumulated during the fed state, such as damaged proteins and injured mitochondria, and recycle their building blocks into new cellular materials.[45]

Fasting also allows your fat cells to release the fat-soluble toxins they store. These then travel to the liver, which detoxifies the stuff and sends it out of the body through bile.

12. Probably increased lifespan

If you fast regularly, but not too often, you may live longer than if you do not fast. In humans, periodic fasting or caloric restriction activates the SIRT1 gene.[46] SIRT1 acts as a "rescue gene" that initiates repair of free radical damage,

---

[45] Mattson MP, Allison DB, Fontana L, et al., "Meal frequency and timing in health and disease," *Proceedings of the National Academy of Sciences of the United States of America* 2014;111(47):16647-16653. doi:10.1073/pnas.1413965111.

[46] Mattson MP, Duan W, Guo Z, op. cit..

prevents premature cell death, increases energy production by mitochondria (cellular power generators), inhibits fat storage, stimulates fat catabolism, and reduces inflammation and oxidative stress.

Animal studies have demonstrated that periodically fasted animals live longer than their non-fasted peers. For example, in 1945, Anton Carlson and Frederick Hoelzel, both from the University of Chicago Department of Physiology, published a report of their experiments with intermittent fasting of rats.[47] They tested the effects of fasting 1 day in 2, 1 day in 3, and 1 day in 4; the rats ate freely, without any restrictions, on non-fast days. The results indicated that for the "average rat" the 1 day in 3 provided the optimum amount of fasting; 1 day in 2 and 1 day in 4 led to early demise for many rats. Among rats fasted 1 day in 3, the average male rat's lifespan increased by 20%, and the average female's by 15%, compared to non-fasted rats. That would translate to a 12 to 20 year gain in lifespan for a human.

In a 1957 Spanish study of elders, those who engaged in alternate day semi-fasting (~50% caloric restriction days alternated with ~50% caloric surplus days) were half as likely to die over a three-year period. Also, those who fasted were in hospital only 123 days, compared to 219 days for those who ate as much as they wanted every day.[48]

---

[47] Carlson AJ, Hoelzel F, "Apparent prolongation of the life span of rats by intermittent fasting," *J Nutr* 1946 March 1;31(3):363-375. <http://jn.nutrition.org/content/31/3/363.extract>

[48] Johnson JB, Laub DR, John S, "The effect on health of alternate day calorie restriction: Eating less and more than needed on alternate days prolongs life," *Medical Hypotheses* 2006;67:209-211. <http://www.johnsonupdaydowndaydiet.com/pdf/ADCR%20JBJ%20MH.pdf>

Members of the Church of Latter Day Saints, or Mormons, practice regular periodic fasting, typically a 24-hour fast once monthly, and they start this habit in children as young as 8 years of age. Research has demonstrated that Mormons who regularly practice this fasting ritual just once monthly have a significantly reduced risk of atherosclerotic heart disease and diabetes.[49]

Thus, it is likely that reduced feeding frequency and increased fasting will reduce your risk for diabetes and heart disease, two of the leading causes of premature death in modern nations. Periodic limited fasting, even just once a month, will therefore very likely give you an opportunity for a longer healthy lifespan.

[49] Horne BD, May HT, Anderson JL, et al., "Usefulness of Routine Periodic Fasting to Lower Risk of Coronary Artery Disease among Patients Undergoing Coronary Angiography," *Am J Cardiology* 2008;102(7):814-819. doi:10.1016/j.amjcard.2008.05.021. <www.ncbi.nlm.nih.gov/pmc/articles/PMC2572991/>

8 How Fasting Affects Human Performance

There exists a common belief that one must or should eat something before engaging in mental or physical activity in order to ensure that you have sufficient energy to complete the task. The idea is that the energy you need for high performance comes from your most recent meal.

This is a myth. A pretty large meal will provide about 1000 kcal. In comparison, after an overnight fasting period of 16-18 hours, the average lean person can have some 1500 to 2000 kcal stored as glycogen (carbohydrate), and at least 37,000 kcal of total energy reserves (glycogen and fat). A meal or snack is a drop in the bucket of your total body energy stores. Further, food intake primarily goes to replenish depleted energy (glycogen and fat) stores, not directly to use for ongoing energy needs.

You will not "run out of energy" for physical or mental activity just 16, 20, 24, 36, or even 48 hours after eating. You would have to go without food for 90 days or more to totally deplete your body's energy reserves.

I once believed that I would be unable to do heavy physical training on an empty stomach, and would make sure that I scheduled my heavy training sessions after meals. However, after learning that my belief was incorrect and experimenting with training in a fasted state, I realized that eating before training had never given me any benefit.

In fact, if it had any effect on my performance at all, it was negative, in the form of stomach cramps or discomfort while working hard, particularly if sprinting, falling and rolling (martial arts), or doing movements that require strong abdominal muscle activation. I have found that I function best in physical training if I do it toward the end of my 16-20 hour overnight fast (which currently is usually in the morning).

You may fear that doing exercise before eating will make you extremely ravenous, but research has shown that doing physical activity in a fasted state has little impact on appetite.[50] This is simply because ongoing physical and mental activities are primarily fueled by your abundant body energy reserves, not by recent food intake. A typical physical exercise session will expend 500 to 1000 kcal, which is only 0.3% of the energy in stored fat and glycogen, a trivial expenditure of energy reserves.

Manufacturers of breakfast foods have claimed that skipping meals will cause poor mental performance, but this has been refuted. In fact, for most people, eating a substantial breakfast tends to impair performance.[51]

---

[50] Rogers PJ, Brunstrom JM, "Appetite and energy balancing," *Physiology & Behavior* 6 April 2016. pii: S0031-9384 (16) 30119-6.

[51] Ibid.

Many people notice feeling sleepy after substantial meals, particularly carbohydrate-rich meals, and some take this to be a sign of some physical imbalance or that carbohydrates are harmful. It is neither. This occurs because digesting meals diverts energy away from the central nervous system and stimulates the rest-and-digest parasympathetic nervous system response. It is natural and expected to feel sleepy after substantial meals, especially if you are already in the fed state (e.g. after lunch). This is why traditional cultures scheduled a siesta after the main mid-day meal.

In any case, eating a substantial meal early in the morning stimulates the parasympathetic nervous response, which tends to make one less alert and quick, both mentally and physically. This effect may be reduced if you have fasted sufficiently and done significant physical activity prior to eating the first meal.

9 IMPLEMENTING PERIODIC FASTING

As already noted, in this manual, fasting means not eating or drinking anything that provides energy (calories). Most people do an absolute fast for at least 10-12 hours overnight. To obtain the benefits of absolute fasting discussed above, it is necessary to extend the daily fasting period to about 16-18 hours, or to fast 24 to 36 hours once or twice weekly, or combine these two approaches.

You might feel intimidated by the idea of fasting 16-18 hours and eating only eating only two meals on a daily basis, even more by the suggestion of one or two 20-24 hour fasts each week, but once you actually try it for several weeks, I think you will want to continue indefinitely.

Ground Rules

During your fasting periods you may consume non-caloric beverages including:
- Water (preferably filtered with a solid carbon block filter)
- Herbal teas
- Green or black tea

I recommend avoiding all beverages sweetened with artificial non-caloric sweeteners. Studies show refined sugar and non-caloric sweeteners have addictive properties, making you want more sweets and sweet flavors in your food. In one study, mice given the choice of unlimited access to cocaine, sugar, or saccharine chose sugar or saccharine over cocaine even if they were previously addicted to cocaine.[52] In addition, we have considerable evidence that eating non-caloric sweeteners stimulate sweets cravings, overeating and weight gain.[53]

One purpose of a fast is to break your addiction to intensely sweetened foods. Generally, limit the use of all non-caloric sweeteners during a fast. However if adding a non-caloric natural sweetener like licorice or stevia to your tea helps you stick to your fast, do that. I recommend drinking water, herbal tea, kukicha (twig tea), roasted green tea, roasted barley tea, or roasted dandelion tea during your fast.

Extending Your Daily Fast

The easiest way to gain the benefits of fasting lies in limiting yourself to two daily meals and fitting all the meals of any day into an "eating window" lasting 6 to 8 hours, thus extending the daily period of continuous fasting to 16 to 18 hours. Here's how to transition to time-restricted feeding:

Step 1: Eliminate snacks

If you've been eating more than 3 times daily, start by cutting out all of your snacks and reducing to not more than 3 meals daily. At the times you would have eaten a snack or snacks, have a non-caloric beverage. If you have been eating only two or three meals daily, move on to step 2.

---

[52] Lenoir M, Serre F, Cantin L, Ahmed SH, "Intense Sweetness Surpasses Cocaine Reward," *PLoS ONE* 2007 ;2(8): e698. doi:10.1371/ journal.pone.0000698

[53] Yang Q, "Gain weight by "going diet?" Artificial sweeteners and the neurobiology of sugar cravings: Neuroscience 2010," *The Yale Journal of Biology and Medicine* 2010;83(2):101-108. <http://www.ncbi.nlm.nih.gov/pmc/articles/PMC2892765/?tool>

Step 2: Identify your optimum daily eating window

As already noted, from a biological standpoint, a significant and growing body of research indicates that humans and some other mammals sustain better metabolic health when they consume most of their food early in their normal waking period (for humans, daylight hours) rather than late in the day.[54, 55, 56] People assigned to consuming the bulk of their food early in the day showed less hunger, greater satiety, lower body fat mass, smaller waist circumference, and lower serum glucose, triglycerides, and insulin levels than those who consumed the bulk of their food late in the day.[57] People who eat late rather than early meals have a higher propensity to gain weight and more difficulty losing it.[58] This occurs because eating during the early part of the

---

[54] Jakubowicz D, Barnea M, et al., "Effects of caloric intake timing on insulin resistance and hyperandrogenism in lean women with polycystic ovary syndrome," *Clinical Science* 2013 Nov 01;125(9):423-432. <http://www.clinsci.org/content/125/9/423.long>

[55] Morgan LM, Shi J-W, et al., "Effect of meal timing and glycaemic index on glucose control and insulin secretion in healthy volunteers," *Br J Nutr* 2012;108:1286-1291.

[56] Jakubowicz D, Barnea M, et al., "High Caloric intake at breakfast vs. dinner differentially influences weight loss of overweight and obese women," *Obesity* 2013 Dec;21(12);2504-2512. <http://onlinelibrary.wiley.com/doi/10.1002/oby.20460/full>

[57] Ibid.

[58] Garaulet M, Gómez-Abellán P, "Timing of food intake and obesity: A novel association," *Physiology & Behavior* 2014 Jul;134:44-50. <http://www.tradewindsports.net/wp-content/uploads/2014/03/Nutrient-Timing-and-Obesity-2014.pdf>

day synchronizes with circadian cycles of hormones and organ functions.[59]

Chinese medicine maintains that all organs have circadian variations in functions. According to Chinese medical theory, the stomach is most receptive to food and most capable of efficient digestion in the hours 7-9 A.M. and weakest in the hours 7-9 P.M.. Biomedical research has confirmed that the stomach empties about 50% more quickly after a meal taken at 8 A.M. compared to a meal taken at 8 P.M.,[60] so food stagnation, indigestion and acid reflux may occur when large meals are taken in the evening rather than the morning. This may also contribute to constipation, as stagnation in the stomach will often impair intestinal peristalsis.

Many people report having no appetite in the morning. I have found that people who lack a morning appetite generally have a habit of eating large meals late in the day. Since late meals are digested inefficiently, you may feel food sitting in your gut when you awaken in the morning. The remedy is quite simple. If one skips or minimizes the last meal of the day, one will generally have a stronger appetite early in the day.

As already noted, some proportion of Seventh Day Adventists eat two meals, generally morning and noon, and SDAs have lower risks of chronic diseases and have a

---

[59] Ibid..

[60] Goo RH, Moore JG, et al., "Circadian Variation in Gastric Emptying of Meals in Humans," *Gastroenterology* 1987;93:515-8.
<http://www.gastrojournal.org/article/0016-5085(87)90913-9/pdf>

greater healthy life expectancy than the average American.[61] Also, for centuries, many Buddhists have followed the traditional discipline (vinaya) to only eat food in the hours between dawn and noon, and fast until dawn after their mid-day meal.

Tracy and I roughly follow this pattern. We are generally up and about, doing meditation, household chores, yoga, martial arts, or strength training, for 2-4 hours before we begin to feel noticeable hunger. We usually eat our first meal sometime between 8 and 10 A.M., after spending 2 to 4 hours in mild to intense physical activity, food preparation, and mental tasks. Then we eat our second meal around 2 P.M. and usually finish by 4 P.M. After the second meal we generally don't feel hungry until about 8 or 10 A.M. the next day, so we find it relatively easy to fast for 16-18 hours daily with very little time spent feeling hunger.

Consider your exercise patterns as well. When you increase your daily fasting period, you will eat larger meals during your eating window and these will take several hours to digest. I don't recommend doing any vigorous physical training within a couple of hours after large meals. We prefer doing our regular resistance and mobility training in the morning before eating, partly because it is more comfortable on an empty stomach, and partly because this prevents us from missing training sessions due to getting involved in other tasks during the day. You may however find that you only have time for exercise in the evening. If so, eating breakfast and lunch but skipping supper may also be the best solution. If you don't eat in the evening, this will

---

[61] Kelly CJ, "A controlled trial of reduced meal frequency without caloric restriction in healthy, normal-weight, middle-aged adults," *Am J Clin Nutr* 2007 Oct; 86(4): 1254-1255.
<http://ajcn.nutrition.org/content/86/4/1254.2.long>

give you time to exercise, several hours after finishing your mid-day meal. Then you can fast until the next morning.

Also consider the timing and quality of your sleep. Due to the fact that the stomach empties more slowly in the evening, taking large meals within three hours of going to sleep can result in restless, dream-filled, unsatisfying sleep. As a general rule, sleep is sounder when the bulk of digestion has been completed by the time one goes to sleep. If you suffer from sleep disturbance, you may want to try having your last large meal finished five or six hours before you go to bed. This will usually result in having an appetite for breaking fast earlier in the next day.

Consider your daytime tolerance for hunger. If you choose to eat your one or two meals in the late afternoon or evening, you may have to endure increasing hunger through your waking hours until your feeding window arrives. As noted above, research shows that people assigned to eat most of their food early in the day reported less hunger and more satisfaction than those assigned to eat most of their food late in the day,[62] and in another study, complaints of daytime hunger were common among individuals who participated in an experiment where they consumed all their food in one 4-hour long evening meal.[63]

By the way, there exists evidence that eating two meals daily is better than one or three. Animals fed two early meals (breakfast and mid-day) had less body weight and fat gain

---

[62] Note 59.

[63] Stote KS, Baer DJ, Spears K, et al., "A controlled trial of reduced meal frequency without caloric restriction in healthy, normal-weight, middle-aged adults," *The Am J Clin Nutr* 2007;85(4):981-988. <http://www.ncbi.nlm.nih.gov/pmc/articles/PMC2645638/>

than those fed either three meals or two late meals, but both groups fed only two meals fared better than the group fed three meals in some metabolic respects.[64] Another study found that animals fed a large breakfast with a smaller supper (two meals daily) fared better than those fed the same amount and type of food in one single daily meal (breakfast only). Those on one meal experienced an increase in body weight gain, elevated blood levels of insulin and leptin, a disturbance of the circadian expression of the Clock gene, and a reduction of gene expression associated with fat oxidation (ß-oxidation) in both fat cells and the liver, in comparison to those eating two meals daily.[65] These adaptations on the one meal daily plan may be predictable: as food income becomes chronically infrequent (i.e. only once every 24 hours), the body may adapt by increasing fat storage (via increased insulin) and reducing fat expenditure to protect against starvation. Thus, for a daily regimen, two meals may produce better health results than either one or three. (Limiting oneself to only one meal on one or two days per week is different because it does not enforce metabolic adaptations to one meal daily; see below.)

If you eat a late breakfast and a main mid-afternoon meal, you will likely feel satisfied all day, through the evening, and spend the longest part of your daily fast asleep. Then, when you awaken, your body will have already shifted overnight into metabolism supported by energy stores (fat and glycogen), which will blunt your morning appetite. Thus you will be able to engage in physical and/or mentally

---

[64] Wu T, Sun L, ZhuGe F, et al., "Differential Roles of Breakfast and Supper in Rats of a Daily Three-Meal Schedule Upon Circadian Regulation and Physiology," *Chronobiology International* 2011 Nov 14;28(10):890-903.

[65] Fuse Y, et al., 2012. Op. cit. (note 29).

challenging activities for at least a couple of hours before you will feel a strong desire to eat. If you wait to eat until later in the day, hunger will arise, and it can be hard to concentrate on other tasks when you feel hungry. We prefer getting our hunger satisfied first, which then frees our attention for our other activities.

Another factor is when to spend time with your family. While many people think of the evening as the time for the family to share a meal, it may not be so. Children of modern families typically have after-school activities that prevent the family from all being together for an evening meal at the same time. Father or mother may be involved in long hours or overtime at work, meetings, chauffeuring children to their activities, volunteering, night school, exercise, or other business. It is often easier for a family to eat together in the morning, before the members disperse in different directions (school, work, etc.). Having a substantial home-cooked meal early in the day also ensures that everyone starts the day off on the right nutritional foot, well-satisfied so less prone to grabbing junk food during the day.

Since the evidence indicates that you will very likely get the best health and fitness results by eating more food in the morning and mid-day and none in the evening, I strongly urge you to adopt this approach. However, I recognize that your experience may vary. If you find that it is more practical for you to have your meal window in the later part of the day, you can still get the benefits of periodic fasting. Just adhere to the principle of fasting about 16-18 hours (give or take a couple of hours) every day.

Step 3: Gradually eliminate the least desired daily meal

One way to gradually get adjusted to longer daily fasting involves doing it one day of your first week of implementation, then add one day each week, so that by the end of 7 weeks you have completely adapted your daily schedule to have a 16-18 hour fast each day. Once you finish this process, if desired you can gradually reduce your eating window from 8 hours to 4-6 hours in the same fashion. The following table illustrates the process I have suggested.

Table 9.1: A possible process for gradually adapting to daily fasting intervals of 16 hours or more.						
Week	Sun.	Mon.	Tues.	Wed.	Thur.	Fri.	Sat.
1	*Fast 16+hrs, eat 2 meals*	Fast 12 hrs—3 meals	Fast 12 hrs—3 meals	Fast 12 hrs—3 meals	Fast 12 hrs—3 meals	Fast 12 hrs—3 meals	Fast 12 hrs—3 meals
2	*Fast 16+hrs, eat 2 meals*	*Fast 16+hrs, eat 2 meals*	Fast 12 hrs—3 meals	Fast 12 hrs—3 meals	Fast 12 hrs—3 meals	Fast 12 hrs—3 meals	Fast 12 hrs—3 meals
3	*Fast 16+hrs, eat 2 meals*	*Fast 16+hrs, eat 2 meals*	*Fast 16+hrs, eat 2 meals*	Fast 12 hrs—3 meals	Fast 12 hrs—3 meals	Fast 12 hrs—3 meals	Fast 12 hrs—3 meals
4	*Fast 16+hrs, eat 2 meals*	*Fast 16+hrs, eat 2 meals*	*Fast 16+hrs, eat 2 meals*	*Fast 16+hrs, eat 2 meals*	Fast 12 hrs—3 meals	Fast 12 hrs—3 meals	Fast 12 hrs—3 meals
5	*Fast 16+hrs, eat 2 meals*	*Fast 16+hrs, eat 2 meals*	*Fast 16+hrs, eat 2 meals*	*Fast 16+hrs, eat 2 meals*	*Fast 16+hrs, eat 2 meals*	Fast 12 hrs—3 meals	Fast 12 hrs—3 meals
6	*Fast 16+hrs, eat 2 meals*	*Fast 16+hrs, eat 2 meals*	*Fast 16+hrs, eat 2 meals*	*Fast 16+hrs, eat 2 meals*	*Fast 16+hrs, eat 2 meals*	*Fast 16+hrs, eat 2 meals*	Fast 12 hrs—3 meals

7	Fast 16+hrs, eat 2 meals	Fast 16+hrs, eat 2 meals	Fast 16+hrs, eat 2 meals	Fast 16+hrs, eat 2 meals	Fast 16+hrs, eat 2 meals	Fast 16+hrs, eat 2 meals	Fast 16+hrs, eat 2 meals

Eat your two daily meals within an 8 hour period or less. For example, eat breakfast between 7 and 10 a.m. and start your last meal 3 to 6 hours after you finish breakfast. Or, eat breakfast at mid-day and finish your last meal 6 hours later. In this way you can arrange a 18 to 20 hour fast each day.

Remember, on days when you have only 2 meals, you can eat to satisfaction of whole plant foods at both of those meals. Fasting regularly generally improves your selection of foods. After you fast a 16 or more hours, you will generally prefer healthy, substantial foods, not junk.

How I Eased Into Daily Fasting

In my case, many years ago, when I first started daily extended fasting, I first eliminated my fourth daily feeding, which was an evening snack about 7 P.M. This made me feel hungrier in the morning, so I started increasing the caloric content of my breakfast.

After some time, I had built up my breakfast to a point that I wanted to move my second meal to a little later time, and I had improved the energy content of lunch to a point that I easily eliminated my late afternoon meal.

That left me with two meals: my breakfast, usually taken between 8 and 10 A.M., and my supper, taken usually between 2 and 3 P.M.. As already noted, following this schedule, I will generally eat breakfast right about when I start feeling hungry; my second meal keeps me full the rest of the day.

Weekly Fasts

Although based on the research cited above I don't consider this optimal, some people may prefer to eat a "normal" 3 meals daily on most days, but fast for 20-24 hours once or twice weekly. This is better than not fasting at all. Others may want to combine daily ~16-18 hour fasts with longer 20-24 hour fasts once or twice weekly.

Fasting 24 hours once or twice weekly is a simple (but not necessarily easy) way to reduce your total energy intake to achieve fat loss, without having to endure hunger every day. Removing one or two meals from one day will reduce your calorie intake by 1000-2000 calories; done twice weekly you will create a caloric deficit that will result in a loss of one-half to one pound of fat weekly.

To fast 24 hours, abstain from food from the last meal of one day to the same time the next day. Based on the data showing that large morning meals produce a greater satiety and less hunger sensation than skipping early meals to only eat a late meal, I would recommend the 24 hour fast be accomplished by eating a substantial early (8-10 A.M.) breakfast, then fasting 24 hours until the same time the next morning. If you finish breakfast at 10 A.M. you would fast until 10 A.M. the next day, at which time you would have a substantial breakfast. Alternatively, you can fast from evening to evening – e.g. from 6 P.M. Monday to 6 P.M. Tuesday – although I think that, due to daytime hunger, you will find this will be much more challenging than fasting from morning to morning.

To fast 36 hours on occasion, abstain from food from the last meal of one day to the morning two days later; for example, from 6 P.M. Friday evening to 6 A.M. Sunday morning.

Limiting oneself to only one meal daily only once or twice weekly will not train the body to increase fat storage and reduce fat oxidation because the 24 hour fasts occur infrequently and interrupted by 3-6 days of regular food intake.

A schedule with 14-hr fasts daily and one 24-hr fast in a week could look like this:

Day	Eating	Fasting
1	8 A.M. – 6 P.M.	6 P.M. D1 – 8 A.M. D2
2	8 A.M. – 6 P.M.	6 P.M. D2 – 8 A.M. D3
3	8 A.M. – 6 P.M.	6 P.M. D3 – 8 A.M. D4
4	8 A.M. – 6 P.M.	6 P.M. D4 – 8 A.M. D5
5	8 A.M. – 6 P.M.	**9 A.M. D5 – 9 A.M. D6**
6 Fast to 9 A.M.	8 A.M. – 6 P.M.	6 P.M. D6 – 8 A.M. D7
7	8 A.M. – 6 P.M.	6 P.M. D7 – 8 A.M. D8

A schedule with two 24-hr fasts in a week could look like this:

Day	Eating	Fasting
1	8 A.M. – 6 P.M.	6 P.M. D1 – 8 A.M. D2
2	8 A.M. – 9 A.M.	**9 A.M. D2 – 9 P.M. D3**
3 Fast to 9 A.M.	9 A.M. – 6 P.M.	6 P.M. D3 – 8 A.M. D4
4	8 A.M. – 6 P.M.	6 P.M. D4 – 8 A.M. D5
5	8 A.M. – 9 A.M.	**9 A.M. D5 – 9 P.M. D6**
6 Fast to 9 A.M.	9 A.M. – 6 P.M.	6 P.M. D6 – 8 A.M. D7
7	8 A.M. – 6 P.M.	6 P.M. D7 – 8 A.M. D8

You can adjust the daily feeding window and fasting period to your preference. For example, you could restrict your daily feeding window to 8 A.M. – 4 P.M. so that you fast 16 hours daily *and* once or twice weekly, extend that fast to 24 hours.

10 FASTING FOR FAT LOSS

In order to lose body fat, you absolutely must create and sustain a negative fat balance, and, unless you are also gaining muscle mass, this negative fat balance must occur in the context of a net energy deficit over a period of time. That is, you must both consume less fat than your body burns, and less total energy than you expend.

Most often people try to cut down on the size of meals, resulting in meal-by-meal calorie counting. This has the drawback of increasing the amount of attention you have to give to planning meals and thinking about what and how much you will eat, which may actually have the undesired effect of stimulating appetite. Further, small meals can tease you, in that you get a little to eat, but not enough to feel satisfied in the moment. This teasing can lead you to eat more when you are trying to eat less.

It is much simpler to simply skip some meals, which reduces your contact with food. Further, when you go longer without eating, you can eat to satisfaction, and get all the pleasure of eating, at the meals you do eat.

Some authors suggest that skipping meals will lead you to overeat at later meals. I believed this myself at one time, but research shows that although people who are assigned to delay eating until noon-time do eat a little more at their mid-day meal[66] than they would if they hadn't skipped breakfast, they do not end up eating more calories than they would normally eat at snacks and supper, and they end up with an overall lower caloric intake which will result in fat loss.[67] However, as discussed in chapter 9, research indicates that for fat loss and health benefits, it is likely far better to skip the evening meal than to skip breakfast.

Many people sabotage their ability to get lean through unrealistic expectations. The human body has rate limiting steps for many processes. As already mentioned, humans evolved in an environment where they had to expend considerable energy to acquire adequate food from a habitat wherein food resources were relatively limited. Any human ancestor who lost fat rapidly during lean seasons would have perished. Ancestors who burned off fat reserves very slowly were more likely to survive tight times and leave healthy children.

---

[66] Its actually just a late break-fast. Remember, breakfast does not mean "early morning meal," it means what it says, and occurs whenever you break-fasting and start eating.

[67] Rogers PJ, Brunstrom JM, "Appetite and energy balancing," *Physiology & Behavior* 6 April 2016. pii: S0031-9384 (16) 30119-6.

Consequently, the human body burns fat reserves conservatively. Research has shown that the maximum rate of fat loss is about 30 kcal per pound of excess body fat per day.[68] This means that if you should not restrict your weekly food energy intake any more than 210 kcal per pound of fat you want to lose. If you restrict your food energy intake more than that, you will automatically lose lean body mass you do not want to lose.

This has several implications. First, as you become leaner, your rate of fat loss declines. Second, as you become leaner, you must gradually adjust your energy intake (per pound of body mass) upward to prevent loss of lean mass (Table 10.1).

Table 10.1: Maximum daily kcal reduction and rate of fat loss possible without loss of lean mass.			
Desired fat loss (lb.)	Maximum daily fat kcal deficit	Maximum weekly weight loss (lb.)	*Minimum* time required to lose (days)
10	300	0.6	117
20	600	1.2	156
30	900	1.8	174
40	1200	2.4	187
50	1500	3.0	194

So if you want to lose body fat, follow these guidelines:

---

[68] Alpert SS, "A limit on the energy transfer rate from the human fat store in hypophagia," *J Theor Biol* 2005 Mar 7;233(1):1-13.

1) To create a negative fat balance, limit your fat and animal protein intake. Eat a whole foods, plant-based diet that supplies about 20% (15-25%) of calories as fat, by consuming moderate amounts (~1-2 ounces daily) of seeds, nuts, and avocados, and limiting yourself to no more than 1-2 teaspoons of free oil in the daily diet.
2) Restrict animal products to no more than 15% of daily energy intake. It is not necessary to eat animal products daily. Use only wild fish or lean game or pastured animal products and limit these to no more than 100 g (3.5 ounce) portions per 1000 calories consumed (Table 10.2).
3) To create the required negative energy balance, reduce the number of times you eat in a day to two – preferably breakfast and mid-day, fast 16 to 18 hours every day, and consider eating only one meal and fasting 20-24 hours on 1-2 days each week.

Table 10.2: General Upper Limits (UL) for Animal Product Consumption Based on Energy Intake[1]

Daily Energy Intake (kcalories)	Animal Product UL (kcalories)	Animal Product UL (g/oz lean MFP)[2]
1500	225	140 g (5 ounces)
2000	300	190 g (7 ounces)
2500	375	235 g (8 ounces)
3000	400	250 g (9 ounces)
3500	525	330 g (12 ounces)

1. Defining upper limit as 15% of calories. 2. Consume only wild caught fish, wild game, or meat from pastured animals fed only the types of foods they would consume in the wild.

11 FASTING AND GAINING LEAN MUSCLE

Intermittent fasting can help you gain muscle without putting on unwanted fat if you have a regular program of high intensity, progressive resistance strength training and understand how to appropriately manage your food intake to ensure adequate energy and protein intake during your feeding windows.

You must regularly perform high intensity resistance training in order to build or retain muscle. The body will not build new muscle tissue or maintain the muscle it already has unless it is required to cope with the type of activity it regularly encounters. Only high intensity training that places a demand on muscle strength – not endurance – can stimulate muscle gains. Your training program must focus on the largest muscles of the body, namely the hips and thighs, upper back, and chest and shoulders, with exercises like squats, pull ups, rows, dips, and overhead presses. I will give detailed resistance training guidelines in another book.

Intermittent fasting can help a person gain lean weight by creating an internal environment that favors efficient food assimilation and the growth and preservation of muscle.

Intermittent fasting greatly improves food assimilation and nutrient utilization during feeding periods. As discussed already, prolonging your daily fasting period favors higher levels of growth hormone production, and growth hormone promotes both fat loss and muscle growth.

FASTING FAVORS LEAN GAINS

When you regularly fast 16-18 hours daily, your body becomes more efficient at utilizing nutrients during your feeding periods. During absolute fasting, the body shifts into a hormonal condition aimed at preserving muscle while burning fat, because in ancient times, one would need to have the muscle to successfully gather food during fasting periods and therefore survive the fast. Once you eat, this muscle preservation system directs the nutrients you consume to the muscular system to prepare for the next fast and food quest.

As previously noted, an 8 week long study compared the effects on people of eating all caloric requirements in just one as opposed to the conventional three meals per day.[69] This study found that the people assigned to fasting 20 hours daily, then eating all of their caloric requirements in only 1 evening meal each day lost an average of 1.4 kg (3 lb.) body mass and 2.1 kg (4.6 lb.) fat mass over the eight weeks, which means that they gained an average of 1.6 lb. lean mass over the study period, with no change in energy intake or exercise habits. If not experimental error, this increase in lean mass may have resulted from increased GH output that occurs during fasting. However, the authors did not determine whether this apparent increase in lean mass consisted of water, glycogen, muscle, organ tissue, or bone, or some combination. Nevertheless, this report indicates that reducing meal frequency does not lead to loss of lean mass, and may promote lean mass gains.

---

[69] Stote KS, Baer DJ, Spears K, et al, "A controlled trial of reduced meal frequency without caloric restriction in healthy, normal-weight, middle-aged adults," *Am J Clin Nutr* 2007;85(4):981-988.
<http://www.ncbi.nlm.nih.gov/pmc/articles/PMC2645638/>

FEASTING FAVORS FAT GAINS

Contrary to common belief, it is not necessary nor beneficial to *continuously* maintain an excess kcaloric intake for weeks on end in order to build muscle. If you have at least 10% body fat, you have plenty of energy reserves to draw upon for fueling muscle growth that occurs after high intensity training sessions. Further, after you sustain an excess caloric intake for more than a few days in a row, the majority of the excess ends up stored as body fat, not muscle mass.

For example, a 140 pound male at 10% body fat carries 14 pounds of fat. About half of that is essential fat that can't be used for energy, so 7 pounds of his body fat is available for energy reserves and provides 24,500 kcalories. A pound of muscle itself is 70% water, and about 30% protein, so it represents the storage of only 136 g of protein and 550 kcal. Hence, a man carrying just 7 pounds of non-essential fat has energy reserves equivalent to the caloric value of nearly 45 pounds of muscle!

Average American men and women have about 28 and 40% body fat, respectively. American men and women with *normal* Body Mass Indices (< 25) have an average body fat of 23 and 34%.[70] Thus, most Americans, including those who may appear lean to the untrained observer, have plenty of excess energy available on their bodies to fuel muscle growth. They do not need to increase their caloric intake for this purpose.

---

[70] St-Onge M-P, "Are Normal-Weight Americans Over-Fat?," *Obesity (Silver Spring, Md)*. 2010;18(11):10.1038/oby.2010.103. doi:10.1038/oby.2010.103.
<http://www.ncbi.nlm.nih.gov/pmc/articles/PMC3837418/#R1>

Table 11.1: Body Fat Percentage Categories		
Category	**Women**	**Men**
Athletes	14-20%	6-13%
Fitness	21-24%	14-17%
Average	25-31%	18-24%
Obese	32%+	25%+

Nor is it necessary to consume extraordinary amounts of protein. To gain 2 pounds of muscle a month, one would add 272 g of protein to one's frame each 30 days, which amounts to only a fraction more than 9 extra grams of protein daily above normal requirements. That can be obtained by taking just one cup of plain unsweetened soy milk or a mere 1 ounce of lean animal flesh daily.

Studies show that overeating does create a hormonal environment that favors some lean tissue gain, but it also favors fat gain over time. About 46% of weight gained by overeating (without concurrent resistance exercise) consists of lean body mass. Over a short-term, research shows that fat and lean mass are gained at approximately the same daily rate during overfeeding.

In one study, subjects who overate 1200-1600 kcal daily gained 4 pounds of lean mass (and 4.7 pounds of fat) over the course of 21 days.[71] While some of this lean gain was muscle the authors did not determined exactly what proportion of the lean gains obtained by overeating consists of increases in intestinal contents, retention of water and storage of glycogen, as opposed to contractile muscle tissue.

Presumably adding resistance exercise would increase the percentage of lean gain, but unless you need to gain some fat due to being too lean, you would probably prefer to avoid gaining fat altogether.

---

[71] Forbes GB, Brown MR, Welle SL, Underwood LE, "Hormonal response to overfeeding," *Am J Clin Nutr* 1989;49:608-11.

Long-term overeating (a high kcalorie diet) in order to "bulk up" may actually reduce your capacity to gain muscle, because it increases fat gain and insulin resistance within days,[72] and obesity and insulin resistance are both associated with increased myostatin expression.[73] Myostatin suppresses muscle growth and insulin resistance impedes protein synthesis. Resistance exercise, aerobic exercise, and body fat loss through caloric restriction all independently reduce expression of myostatin.[74] Thus, overeating actually counteracts the myostatin-reducing (muscle-building) effects of resistance exercise, while staying lean through modest increases in caloric intake probably increases your ability to gain muscle by reducing expression of myostatin.

---

[72] Boden G, Homko C, Barrero CA, et al., "Excessive caloric intake acutely causes oxidative stress, GLUT4 carbonylation, and insulin resistance in healthy men," *Sci Transl Med*. 2015;7(304).

[73] Allen DL, Hittel DS, McPherron AC, "Expression and Function of Myostatin in Obesity, Diabetes, and Exercise Adaptation," *Medicine and science in sports and exercise*. 2011;43(10):1828-1835. doi:10.1249/MSS.0b013e3182178bb4. <https://www.ncbi.nlm.nih.gov/pmc/articles/PMC3192366/>

[74] Ryan AS, Li G, Blumenthal JB, Ortmeyer HK, "Aerobic Exercise+Weight Loss Decreases Skeletal Muscle Myostatin Expression and Improves Insulin Sensitivity in Older Adults," *Obesity (Silver Spring, Md)*. 2013;21(7):1350-1356. doi:10.1002/oby.20216. <https://www.ncbi.nlm.nih.gov/pmc/articles/PMC3742694/>

Thus the fact that you gain weight and some lean mass during overeating does not necessarily indicate that the overeating itself is responsible for adding significant muscle mass to the body. If overeating was a potent method for muscle growth, one could become a powerful strength athlete simply by overeating. We all know this does not happen. The body only adds muscle tissue if it is required to adapt to the types of demands you regularly impose upon it.

GAINING BY TRAINING: SLOW BUT SURE

Many people try overeating to boost their rate of muscle growth because they mistakenly believe that typical trainees can gain muscle at rapid rates, such as 1-2 pounds of muscle per week. Research shows that typical individuals in intensive resistance training will only gain on average 1-2 pounds of muscle *per month* – that's only one-quarter to one-half pound of muscle per week – when complete novices, with a wide variation between individuals, and then the rate of gain tapers considerably as strength gains slow down and the quest to gain muscle requires more patience and persistence over a long term.[75, 76]

Consider that if you did gain one pound of muscle per week, this would amount to 52 pounds of gain in a year. That would transform the typical 5'10" tall, 154 pound male into a 206 pound individual comparable to an elite bodybuilder. Yet not even elite bodybuilders – who are all of relatively rare genetic stock – gain muscle at this rate.

---

[75] Pilon B, *How Much Protein?* (Strength Works, 2008-2009): 39.

[76] Cureton KJ, et al., "Muscle hypertrophy in men and women," *Medicine and Science in Sports and Exercise* 1988; 20(4): 338-344.

To illustrate: Over his 15 year career, 9-time Mr. Olympia Dorian Yates, a genetically gifted and drug-assisted bodybuilder, gained a total of 70 pounds, an average gain of less than 5 pounds per year. Yates gained more per year in the earlier stages and less later, but this illustrates how difficult it is to gain muscular body mass, even for the genetically gifted. In short, if you were to gain 5 pounds of muscle in a year – less than half a pound of muscle per month – you would be matching the average rate of muscle gain found in elite bodybuilders who use anabolic steroids.

Therefore, in reality most people only need *at most* 550-1100 extra kcalories and 136-272 extra grams of protein *per month* – that's only 20-40 kcalories and 5-9 g protein per day – to sustain genetically typical rates of muscle growth. If you want to add 20-30 pounds of muscle to your body, count on taking 2-4 years or more to accomplish it unless you are genetically gifted with unusually low myostatin levels (and/or using anabolic pharmaceuticals).

To reiterate, muscle only grows in response to an imposed demand for an increase in strength (force production capacity), so the most important thing for muscle gain is progressive resistance exercise. Any change in muscle mass produced by altering what, when, or how much you eat is of minor significance in comparison to adaptation to progressive resistance exercise. That means consistent, persistent training that involves a sustainable, gradual significant increase in the resistance against which you exert your force.

MEAL TIMING AROUND TRAINING

So long as your energy and protein intake is overall adequate to support muscle growth, the timing of the meals in relation to training is of secondary importance. The key dietary step is to eat a large, protein- and energy-rich meal within 3-4 hours on either side (before or after) doing your high intensity resistance training.

This meal should contain at least 20 g protein if you are young, and at least 40 g of protein if you are elderly (elders show a blunted response to only 20 g protein).[77] If you train in the morning on an empty stomach, eat your meal within a few hours of finishing training. If you train in the evening, have the meal either a few hours before or shortly after the training session.

If you complete your training session within 3-4 hours of an adequate previous meal, there is a lack of evidence that eating immediately after a training session is necessary to obtain maximum gains from a resistance training session.[78] Thus, if you eat morning and midday meals, you can train before breakfast, between the two meals, or 3-4 hours after the second meal, and in the latter case, do not need to take a post-training meal because nutrients available from the midday meal will be sufficient.

---

[77] Aragon A, Schoenfeld BJ, "Nutrient timing revisited: is there a post-exercise anabolic window?," *J Int Soc Sports Nutr* 2013 Jan 29;10:5 <https://jissn.biomedcentral.com/articles/10.1186/1550-2783-10-5>

[78] Ibid.

If you cannot start training until 5-6 hours after the midday meal, simply increase the energy and protein content of the midday meal; larger meals take longer to digest and create a longer post-meal anabolic window. If instead you eat a midday and evening meal (not ideal), again you can train before the breakfast, between the two meals, or after the evening meal.

EATING FOR MUSCLE GAINS

If you are already lean, you may need only a small increase in total food intake on days of intense exercise. If you are not already in the lean category, you can maintain energy balance or deficit. If you can arrange your schedule for the purpose, you can take advantage of the anabolic effect of training by slightly increasing your energy and protein intake in the meal you consume before or after your training sessions.

For example, let's say your maintenance energy intake is 2500 kcal, and you do resistance training on Monday, Wednesday, and Friday. On Monday, Wednesday, and Friday you eat 2800 kcal in your 4-8 hour feeding window, and at least half of this is consumed within two hours following your training session. On Tuesday and Thursday you consume 2250, and on Saturday and Sunday you consume 2500 kcal. On Monday you start the cycle over. This calorie-cycling program is depicted in table 11.2.

Table 11.2: Example of a Possible Caloric Cycling Schedule to Promote Muscle Gains (assuming 2500 kcal maintenance requirements)

Day	Caloric Intake
1 Resistance Training	2800
2	2250
3 Resistance Training	2800
4	2250
5 Resistance Training	2800
6	2500
7	2500

Over the seven days, you will have taken an excess of 300 kcal on three days, sustained a deficit of 250 kcal on two days, and eaten a maintenance level on two days, so your net excess is about 400 kcal, about the amount needed for the addition of a pound of muscle per week. In addition, you have taken the excess kcalories primarily on the days you trained, ensuring that they would go primarily to the promotion of lean weight gain, rather than fat stores; and you have fasted 16-20 hours on all days. You get all the health benefits of longer fasting periods, while also sustaining a very slight caloric excess to support lean weight gain.

This level of energy surplus may be excessive and promote unwanted fat gain. As discussed above, most people will not gain a pound of muscle per week for very long, if at all. However, it could be too little for some people as well. If you aren't gaining 1-2 pounds per month, slightly increase the surplus caloric intake on training days.

According to the plan above, on resistance training days you would consume about 200-300 excess kcalories in your feeding window. One easy way to do this without feeling stuffed and losing your appetite would be to maintain your normal size meals, but add a 200-300 kcal liquid containing 9-15 g protein – e.g. 2 cups of soymilk – to be consumed in the few hours after your training session, on top of the post-training break-fast meal. Liquids are generally less satiating than solid food, making them ideal for adding energy to the diet without making you so full that it impairs your appetite for your regular meals.

If after adding liquid calories to your diet for a month or two you notice significant fat gain, you may want to reduce the caloric content. Probably most people only need to add one cup of soymilk, since that provides about 100 calories and 8 grams of protein, more than enough to support the typical rate of muscle gain.

To reiterate, one should focus on hard, progressive training, and if you do that you can generally let your appetite guide your food intake, because hard training that makes a demand for new muscle will generally increase your appetite a bit. Eat more only if you are hungry for more, not if you're not.

Since gaining muscle is likely inhibited by continuous overeating and simultaneous gaining of fat tissue, but is supported by efficient assimilation and use of nutrients, and by reducing insulin resistance and myostatin expression, all of which are facilitated by periodic fasting, periodic fasting can help you gain muscle without gaining fat you don't want, provided you engage in regular, progressive resistance training.

12 BREAKING FAST: WHAT TO EAT

Contrary to popular belief, brief fasting (16-36 hours) does not weaken the digestive system or make it necessary to only gradually reintroduce solid foods. On the contrary, after a fast of this length, you will have a strong appetite (a sign of a strong digestive system) and prefer and require substantial foods. Breaking a fast with a puny meal will only leave you unsatisfied.

Make sure your break-fast meals are substantial and nutrient-dense. Whole cereals, legumes, seeds, fruits and vegetables are the best foods to consume post-fasting, as they provide sufficient caloric and nutrient density to quickly satisfy your post-fast appetite without being so calorically dense that you will wipe out the fat-burning benefits of the fasting.

Since we obtain a large proportion of our water requirements from foods we eat, it can be beneficial to break your fasts with warm liquids, such as the teas mentioned in the previous section, or to include a porridge or soup in your break-fast meal. However, this is not required.

It is also desirable to consume a portion of starchy food that supplies at least 100 g of carbohydrate in the break-fast meal to replenish liver glycogen. Replenishing liver glycogen will ensure that your brain gets adequate glucose during your waking hours.

Since both fasting and high intensity exercise improve your muscle uptake of glucose and amino acids, the break-fast meal is an also an excellent opportunity to replenish muscle glycogen and provide protein for muscle repair and growth, especially if you have exercised intensely (resistance training, sprinting, hill climbing) prior to breaking the fast.

Include a substantial portion of plant protein – beans, peas, lentils, or tofu – in the break-fast meal. These foods quickly satisfy hunger, and beans, peas, and lentils stabilize blood sugar levels for many hours, even overnight until the next meal.[79]

Here is a recipe for a substantial porridge, suitable for breakfast in cooler seasons and regions, combining whole cereals, legumes, seeds, and vegetables:

3/4 cup lentils or mung beans
3/4 cup steel cut oats   *+ flax seeds*
_ 3/4 cup millet   *or black sesame*
1/4 cup sunflower or pumpkin seeds
1/4 cup dried cranberries or goji berries
1/4 cup raisins or 3-4 jujube or deglet dates
1-2 cups kabocha, butternut, or buttercup squash or 1 whole sweet potato, peeled and chopped
8 cups filtered water
1/2 tsp unrefined sea salt

---

[79] Greger M, "Beans and the Second Meal Effect," *NutritionFacts.org* 2013 July 5, Volume 13.
<http://nutritionfacts.org/video/beans-and-the-second-meal-effect/>

Soak the legumes and cereal grains in the water overnight. At the appropriate time, bring these to a boil (do not replace the water). After the whole has been brought to a full boil for 5 minutes, add the salt. Turn down the heat. If using a gas stove, put a flame tamer between the pot and the flame, and let it all simmer on low to medium low for 45 minutes to an hour.

Top with 1-2 tablespoons of freshly ground flax seeds or black sesame seeds.

This provides two servings, each providing about 900 kcalories, 147 g carbohydrate, 43 grams of protein, and abundant vitamins and minerals without the additional seeds on top.[80]

One of my favorite post-training break-fasts in the warmer months consists of a bowl of Quick Prep Oats with a side of grilled or :

1.5 cup rolled oats
2-4 tablespoons dried cranberries or goji berries
1 tablespoon ground flaxseed
1.5 cup boiling water
pinch of salt

2 tablespoons peanut or almond butter *or* 1/4 cup peanuts or almonds

1/4 to 1/2 block of firm tofu, grilled or steamed
2 cups mixed vegetables (e.g. broccoli, carrots, summer squash)
1 peach, nectarine, or other seasonal fruit of similar size

---

[80] About one-half the daily requirements for an average individual.

Add the salt to the oats, flax and cranberries or goji berries in a heat-proof bowl. Pour the boiling water over those ingredients and mix thoroughly. Place saucer as a lid over the top of the bowl and let this sit for at least one hour up to overnight. When ready to eat, add the nut butter and stir thoroughly.

Grill the tofu or steam it with the vegetables.[81] Have the fruit before or after the cereal, tofu, and vegetables.

This meal provides up to 1150 kcals, about 126 g carbohydrate, 57 g protein, and 42 g fat, and plenty of vitamins and minerals as well.

When you are not fasting, base your diet on the following foods:
- Whole grains, including
  - Legumes and legume products, particularly lentils, chickpeas, adukis (adzukis), black beans, peas, peanuts, and soy beans
  - Cereals and whole cereal products (such as noodles and breads), including brown rice, barley, wheat, corn, rye, buckwheat, oats, teff, quinoa, amaranth, sorghum, and others
  - Seeds such as sunflower, sesame, flax, hemp, chia, pumpkin, and others
- Seasonal vegetables, including
  - Roots and tubers, like carrots, turnips, burdock, radishes, sunchokes, sweet potatoes, and others
  - Stems, like scallions, leeks and celery
  - Bulbs, like onions and garlic

---

[81] Recipes in ESSENTIAL MACROBIOTICS and BASIC MACROBIOTIC MENUS & RECIPES. See Additional Reading section below.

- Leaves, like bok choy, cabbage, collards, kale, mustard greens, and others
- Flowers, like broccoli and cauliflower
- Fruits, like cucumbers, summer squashes, winter squashes, tomatoes, and others
- Sea vegetables including kelp, dulse, nori, alaria, wakame, hijiki, arame, sea palm, ocean ribbons, and others
- Fresh locally grown seasonal fruits
- Small amounts of nuts (generally, 1-2 ounces daily)
- Small amounts of lean fish or meat from wild or pasture-fed animals (no more than 15% of total energy intake) *or* supplements of vitamin B12 and omega-3 fats (DHA and EPA)

To learn more about how to eat when you are not fasting, get copies of our other books:

ESSENTIAL MACROBIOTICS: THE UNIVERSAL WAY OF SELF-REALIZATION

THE MACROBIOTIC ACTION PLAN: YOUR MAP TO GREATER HEALTH & HAPPINESS

BASIC MACROBIOTIC MENUS & RECIPES.

ADDITIONAL READING

Johnson JB, Laub DR. The Alternate-Day Diet: Turn on Your "Skinny Gene," Shed the Pounds, and Live a Longer and Healthier Life. Perigree Books, 2009.

Matesz D. Powered By Plants: How Natural Selection Adapted Humans to a Whole Foods Plant-Based Diet. Integrity Press and Create Space Publishing Platform, 2013, 2016.

Matesz D and Matesz T. Essential Macrobiotics: The Universal Way of Self-Realization. Integrity Press and Create Space Publishing Platform, 2016.

Matesz T. The Macrobiotic Action Plan. Integrity Press and Create Space Publishing Platform, 2016.

Matesz T and Matesz D. Basic Macrobiotic Menus & Recipes. Integrity Press and Create Space Publishing Platform, 2016.

Pilon B. Eat Stop Eat. Strength Works, Inc., 2010.

Pilon B. How Much Protein? Strength Works, Inc., 2008-2009.

Mattson MP, Allison DB, Fontana L, et al. Meal frequency and timing in health and disease. Proceedings of the National Academy of Sciences of the United States of America. 2014;111(47):16647-16653. doi:10.1073/pnas.1413965111.

Trepanowski JF, Bloomer RJ. The impact of religious fasting on human health. Nutrition Journal. 2010;9:57. doi:10.1186/1475-2891-9-57.

Printed in Great Britain
by Amazon